J.D. RODRIGUEZ

Bodybuilding and Nutrition Fundamental's

It may not be for you, but this 12-Week Guide to Build Muscle and Lose Fat is the Best for Beginners.

This book was professionally typeset on Reedsy.
Find out more at reedsy.com

Contents

1

Introduction

"*Success is not final, failure is not fatal: It is the courage to continue that counts." — Winston Churchill.*

For the past 15 years I've been OBSESSED with one thing and one thing only... getting my physique to a level that I was proud of. I got certified as a personal trainer and nutrition coach and I even had my own coaching side hustle for a little bit. I'm writing this book for the person that is just starting their bodybuilding journey and give them the knowledge I wish I had when I first started. But why should you listen to me?? I'm just a guy that figured out how to build muscle with barely any money and through trial and error. A LOT of errors. Hoping you don't make those same mistakes.

In this book you can expect the techniques and ideas that will help you build muscle, lose fat and be able to look yourself in the mirror and be proud of your progress. You will be an example to your family, your friends, and show them that a healthier lifestyle is possible.

You will become an "inspiration" for the people that matter most to you and to other people out and about. Even if you don't speak to them directly, your hard work will speak for itself.

Before we get started here are some people that I would like to mention because I believe they will be helpful to you in this journey that you are about to embark on. Whether you want a better physique, just want to increase your confidence, just want to drop a few pounds and/or increase your knowledge here they are:

- Joe Bennet (Youtube: Hypertrophy Coach)
- Dr. Mike Israetel (Youtube: Renaissance Periodization)
- Dr. Sokolowski (IG: @dr_soko)
- Dr. Christle Guevarra (IG: @dr.christle)
- Dr. Layne Norton (IG: @biolayne)

I would strongly recommend starting with Dr. Mike at Renaissance Periodization. Look for the playlist tab and search for the "**Healthy Eating Made Simple**" and "**Hypertrophy Made Simple**." Those are some great resources.

And if you want to stay away from the false information and make decisions on sound data and science, Layne Norton debunks all the myths and latest claims from other people in the fitness industry and gives you the truths and how you can get a healthier lifestyle.

2

Staying Motivated: Know Your Why

"Success is the sum of small efforts, repeated day in and day out." — Robert Collier

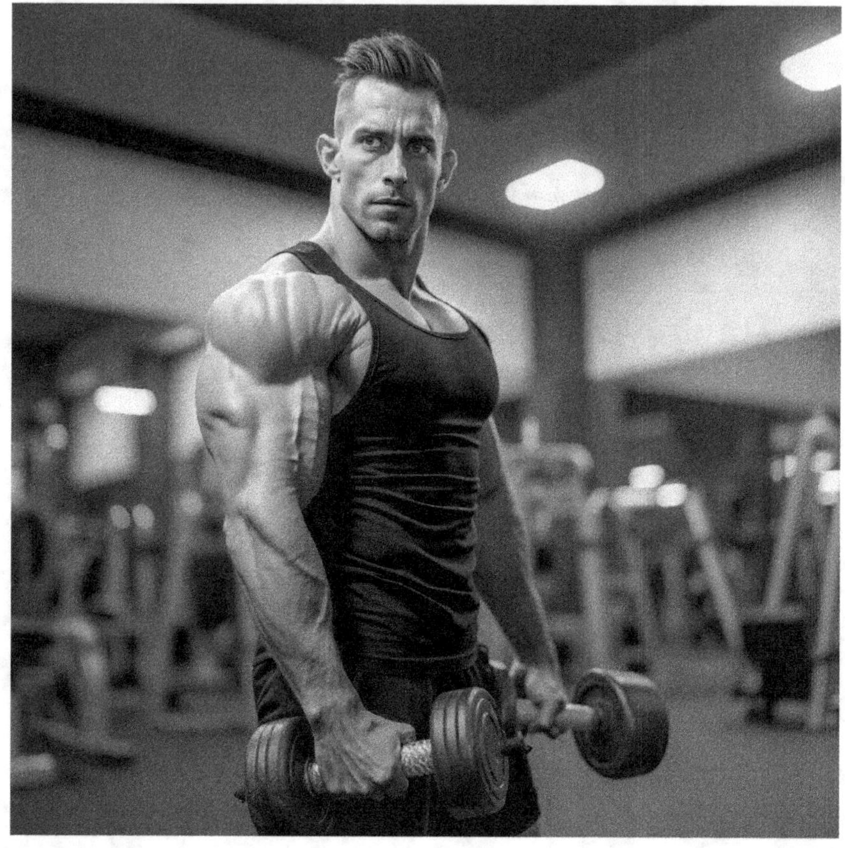

Before you get started with any goal it is important to ask ourselves "Why do I want this?"

Listen, things will come up and challenges will come up. It's a part of life. Your motivation will decrease at some point and your why is going to be the reason that keeps pushing you forward.

Your why is personal to you. Nobody else will be able to understand it better than yourself. Not your parents, not your wife, not your husband, not anybody.

So how do you create a compelling why?

The most important factor is that it has to be emotional. If it brings tears into your eyes the better.

Here's an exercise that I like to do that I got from Dean Graziosi.

Let's say you want to lose 100 pounds in a year. Ask yourself "why do i want to lose 100 pounds in a year?"

Once you get the first answer, ask yourself again "why."

And then keep going for 7 more times or as long as you get an emotional response from the heart.

Why do all this? Because oftentimes our first response is not the real answer. It's the answer that other people want to hear, not your own.

You're only a victim of 3 things... Avoid them!

Most of the time the 3 things that will stop people from achieving their fitness goals are:

- **Your own ignorance**: it's okay to not know what you don't know, but to stay ignorant is not. You can find the answer to whatever question you have on the web. It's much simpler than you think. Especially now with Artificial Intelligence (AI), you can ask ChatGPT a question and will give the answer in a few seconds.

- **Your laziness**: if you're not willing to put in the work, you're not going to get what you want. It's that simple.

- **Your poor decision making**: You can control your life. You can control the food you eat, the information you take in, the people you listen to, etc. you are in control. Don't let anybody tell you otherwise.

3

How Muscles Grow: Where Science and Savagery Meet

"Hard work beats talent when talent doesn't work hard." — *Tim Notke*

The fitness community is riddled with myths and people talking dookie about one another trying to prove who's right and who's wrong. It's pretty annoying and while I'm not going to break down all the science because that will take forever, I will tell you what you need to focus on to make progress.

There are 3 main ways that muscle grow:

- **Muscle Tension**: also known as progressive overload. To achieve this you have to provide stress to muscle that it is not used to in order to adapt and grow. For example: if you did 100 pounds on bench press in one session for 6 repetitions, the following session you can do 105 pounds for 6 repetitions. In simpler terms, lift heavier weights each session for a particular body part or muscle.

- **Muscle Damage**: if you have been sore after a workout then you have experienced muscle damage. However, you do not need to feel sore after every workout to make sure you are growing muscle. As long as you keep providing enough stress/stimulus by progressive overloading the muscle you will grow.

- **Metabolic Stress**: also known as Sarcoplasmic Hypertrophy. People refer to this as the "pump", which causes swelling around the muscle to help it grow without necessarily increasing the size of the muscle cell. This is why you may look bigger while you workout.

This opinion is biased, but I still think it's important. Intensity and focus will be your biggest assets when it comes to building muscle and losing fat. You can have the best workout routine but without intensity (the ability to work hard) and focus (avoid distractions) your result will be mediocre at best.

This is where science and savagery meet… hard work and applied knowledge will take you far in your journey.

4

5 Training Principles

"Discipline is the bridge between goals and accomplishment." – *Jim Rohn*

Before I jump in, all the principles I'm about to share are important. I don't know, but for some reason when you give people a list they always think that the first one is the most important and the last one is the least important. Don't make that assumption.

Principle 1: Mindset

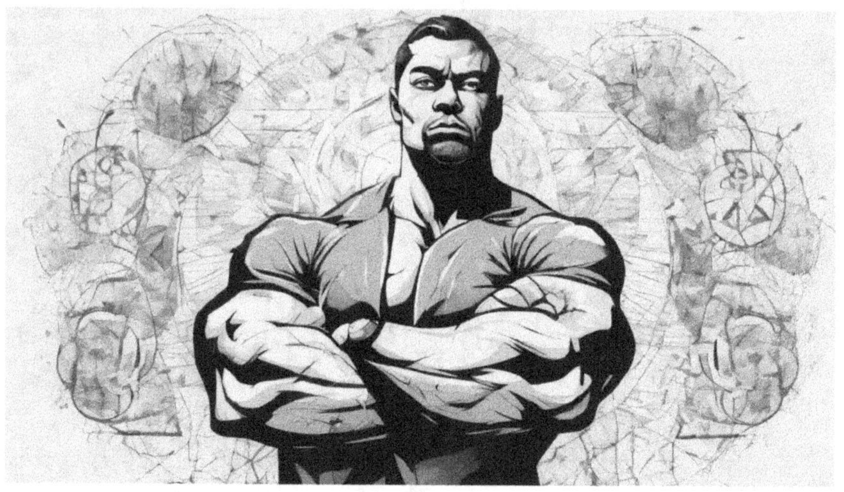

One of my favorite quotes that I recently heard is "I can always learn more, I can always do better, and I can always do more."

Your ability to adapt to a growth mindset will determine how much success in your fitness journey you will have. Of course it will depend on your goals. But if you're someone that is trying to take their physique as far as possible, what works today, may not work for you tomorrow. The fitness industry is always adapting and with new research coming out, there will be better ways to do things. But, like I mentioned before, there is no perfect plan so don't fall into the trap of trying to learn everything before you take action. That is paralysis by analysis. Your best teacher will be the feedback you get from applying what you learn and failure along the way.

Building physical strength is only half of the journey in bodybuilding. Mental resilience and a strong mindset are equally crucial. Here are some tips to develop the mental side of your journey:

- **Stay Positive**: Challenges will come — focus on your progress and don't dwell on setbacks.

- **Visualize Success**: Picture your end goals to stay motivated through tough workouts.

- **Cultivate Discipline**: Motivation may fade, but consistency and discipline will carry you forward.

- **Embrace the Process**: Enjoy the small wins in your journey, such as mastering a new exercise or achieving a personal record.

- **Seek Guidance**: Find a mentor or coach who can help you stay on track and boost your confidence during moments of doubt.

Remember, a positive and focused mindset not only helps with gym performance but also nurtures long-term growth.

Principle 2: Manage Recovery: The Big 3

Sleep

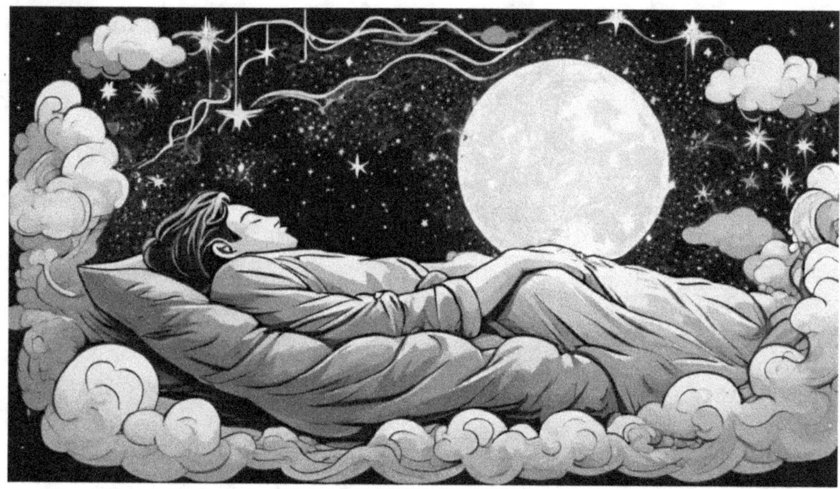

Believe it or not, muscle doesn't grow in the gym. It grows when your recovery is on point. This is why you need to get 8 hrs of sleep every night or more if it's possible.

At the very least, try to get 7 hours of sleep every night.

This how sleep helps you build muscle:

- Increasing production of IGF-1 (insulin-like growth factor 1) and testosterone, which are responsible for muscle growth.

- Stimulating protein synthesis through the release of human growth hormone (HGH).

- Replenishing muscle glycogen stores, allowing for better workout performance.

- Regulating hormones essential for muscle repair and growth.

- Reducing inflammation and promoting muscle relaxation.

Stress

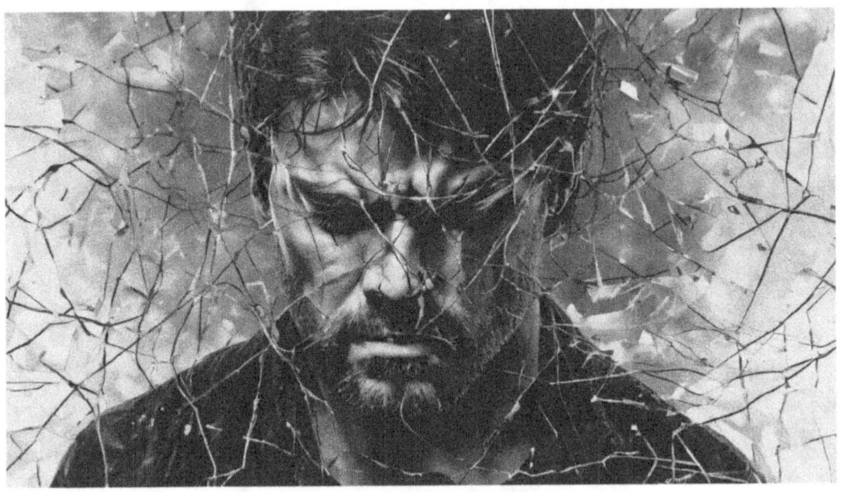

Another important aspect is stress. Life is stressful and it throws curveballs at you. Here's a few ways stress can hinder your muscle building journey:

- **Hormonal Imbalance**: chronic stress elevates cortisol levels, a hormone that can prevent muscle protein synthesis and promote muscle breakdown instead. This imbalance can hinder recovery.

- **Increase fatigue**: high stress levels can lead to mental and physical fatigue, making it difficult to maintain an effective workout routine and reduce motivation, further hindering your journey. Not to mention this can also impact other areas of your life like work, love life, relationships, family, and health.

- **Nutrition**: Stress can affect appetite and food choices, leading to poor nutrition. Adequate protein intake and balanced nutrition are essential for muscle repair and growth.

- **Recovery**: Stress can interfere with sleep quality. Poor sleep affects recovery, which is crucial for muscle growth as this is when repair and growth primarily happen.

In your daily life, high stress levels can affect you in several ways such as:

- **Mental Health**: Stress can contribute to anxiety and depression, affecting overall well-being, motivation, and focus in daily tasks.

- **Physical Health**: Chronic stress can lead to health issues such as high blood pressure, heart disease, and weakened immune function, impacting overall quality of life.

- **Social Relationships**: Stress can strain relationships due to irritability or withdrawal, leading to isolation or conflict with friends and family.

- **Work Performance**: Stress can decrease productivity and focus, leading to mistakes, missed deadlines, and decreased job satisfaction.

Another aspect of stress that is not talked about enough is that chronic stress can kill you. Now, before I tell you how I will say that stress is a natural response and it's not always bad. Unmanageable high stress levels are bad (chronic stress).

According to the American Psychological Association, short-term stress affects all systems including:

- Musculoskeletal (ie., muscle tightening and tension)
- Respiratory (ie., rapid breathing or shallow breathing)

- Cardiovascular(ie., heart race increase, blood pressure increase)
- Endocrine, gastrointestinal, nervous, and reproductive: stress hormone release, flight or fight response

A 2021 research review

Trusted Source

demonstrated the following diseases and illnesses are directly associated with chronic stress:

- anxiety
- depression
- pain
- fatigue

Chronic stress is associated with the following health conditions:

- heart disease and dysfunction (heart attack)
- digestive disorders
- memory disorders
- diabetes
- cancer (particularly breast tumor)

With everything in our society being so high paced, managing our stress levels is a skill that we need to develop for our well-being and longevity. Things like proper nutrition, exercise, mindfulness, gratitude and relaxation can help you manage your stress levels and have a higher quality of life.

If you are experiencing high stress levels seek professional help and explore stress-management techniques.

Nutrition

Nutrition plays a critical role in muscle growth by providing the necessary building blocks (like protein) for muscle repair and growth, energy for workouts (carbohydrates and fats), and essential vitamins and minerals for recovery and overall body functions. Protein is essential for muscle repair and synthesis, while carbohydrates provide energy to fuel workouts. Consuming a diet rich in nutrients and maintaining a calorie surplus of 10% of total calories (if aiming to gain muscle) ensures proper muscle development without putting on excess fat.

How to get your macros and track your calories?

This is a very important aspect because tracking your macros and your calories provides a baseline for which to make further decisions on. Because if you have no data to make decisions on, chances are your progress will be limited.

I like to think of this as a financial budget. Tracking your calories and your macros is a nutritional budget.

Before we get started on tracking your calories let me give you some basic information on carbs, fats and protein.

Carbohydrates (Carbs)

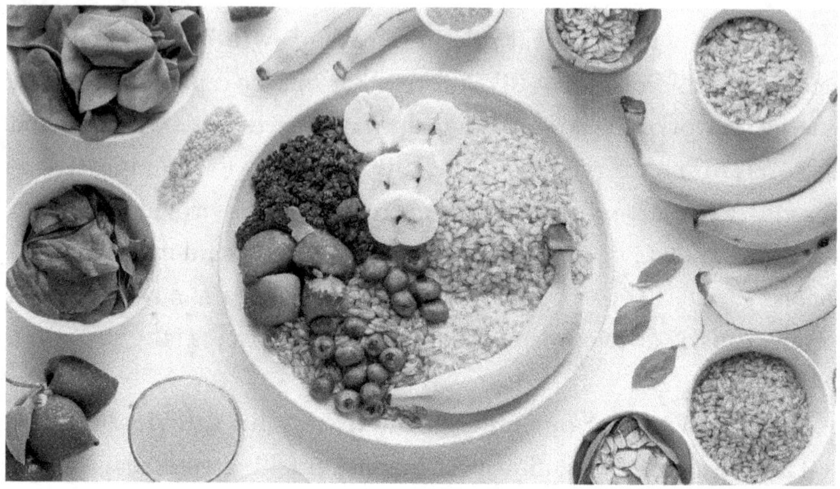

Carbohydrates are one of the three macronutrients that provide energy to the body and there are two type of carbs:

- **Simple Carbohydrates**: These are sugars that are quickly absorbed by the body, providing rapid energy. Examples include glucose, fructose (found in fruits), and sucrose (table sugar).

- **Complex Carbohydrates**: These consist of longer chains of sugar molecules and take longer to digest, providing sustained energy. Examples include whole grains, legumes, and starchy vegetables.

Carbohydrates play several crucial roles in muscle building and performance:

- **Energy Source**: Carbohydrates are the body's primary source of energy, especially during high-intensity exercise. They are stored in the muscles and liver as glycogen, which can be quickly converted to glucose when needed. <u>One gram of carbs equals 4 calories.</u>

- **Glycogen Storage**: Adequate carbohydrate intake helps replenish glycogen stores after workouts. This is essential for recovery and preparing for subsequent training sessions. Low glycogen levels can lead to fatigue and decreased performance.

- **Protein Sparing**: Consuming enough carbohydrates can help spare protein from being used as an energy source. This allows protein to be utilized primarily for muscle repair and growth rather than energy production.

- **Insulin Response**: Carbohydrates stimulate the release of insulin, a hormone that plays a key role in muscle growth. Insulin helps transport glucose and amino acids into muscle cells, promoting recovery and muscle protein synthesis.

- **Enhanced Performance**: Carbohydrates can improve endurance and performance during workouts, allowing for longer and more intense training sessions, which are critical for muscle growth.

Fats

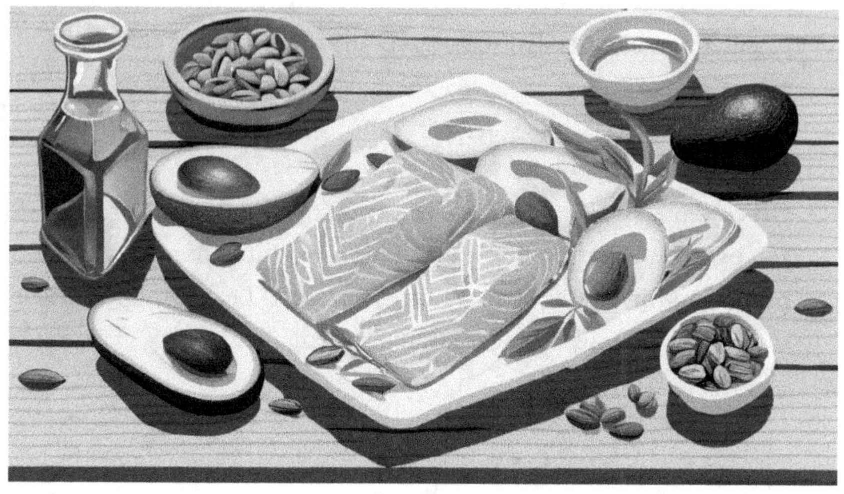

Fatas, also known as lipids, provide energy and support various bodily functions and we have 3 types of fats:

- **Saturated Fats**: Typically solid at room temperature, these fats are found in animal products (like meat and dairy) and some plant oils (like coconut oil). They should be consumed in moderation.

- **Unsaturated Fats**: These are usually liquid at room temperature and are considered healthier. They can be further divided into:

- **Monounsaturated Fats**: Found in olive oil, avocados, and nuts.

- **Polyunsaturated Fats**: Found in fatty fish, flaxseeds, walnuts, and sunflower oil. This category includes omega-3 and omega-6 fatty acids, which are essential for health.

- **Trans Fats**: These are artificially created fats found in some processed foods. They are associated with negative health effects and should be avoided.

Fats play several important roles in muscle building and overall health:

- **Energy Source**: Fats provide a concentrated source of energy, offering 9 calories per gram, which is more than double that of carbohydrates and proteins. This makes them essential for fueling prolonged, low to moderate-intensity exercise.

- **Hormone Production**: Fats are crucial for the production of hormones, including testosterone and other anabolic hormones that play a significant role in muscle growth and recovery.

- **Nutrient Absorption**: Certain vitamins (A, D, E, and K) are fat-soluble, meaning they require fat for proper absorption. These vitamins are important for overall health and can indirectly support muscle function and recovery.

- **Cell Membrane Integrity**: Fats are essential components of cell membranes, including muscle cells. Healthy fats help maintain the structure and function of these membranes, which is vital for muscle contraction and overall cellular health.

- **Inflammation Control**: Omega-3 fatty acids, a type of polyunsaturated fat, have anti-inflammatory properties that can help reduce muscle soreness and promote recovery after intense workouts.

A general guideline is: 20-35% of total daily calories should come from fats, with an emphasis on unsaturated fats.

Protein

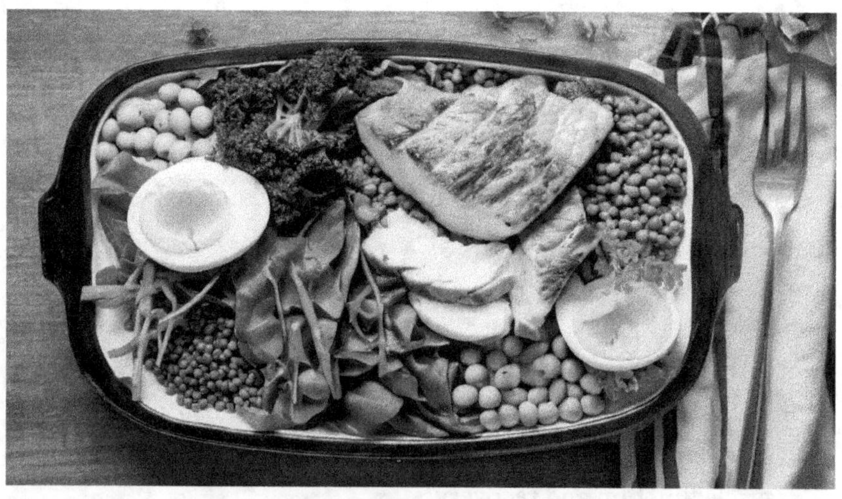

Proteins play a crucial role in various bodily functions, including muscle growth, repair, and overall health. They can be classified based on their source and structure:

- **Animal Proteins**: These are derived from animal products and are considered complete proteins because they contain all nine essential amino acids. Examples:
- Meat (beef, pork, lamb)
- Poultry (chicken, turkey)
- Fish and seafood
- Eggs
- Dairy products (milk, cheese, yogurt)

- **Plant Proteins**: These come from plant sources and may be incomplete proteins, meaning they lack one or more essential amino acids. However, some plant proteins are complete, such as:
- Quinoa
- Soy products (tofu, tempeh, edamame)
- Chia seeds
- Buckwheat
- Certain legumes (lentils, chickpeas, black beans)

- **Protein Supplements**: These include protein powders derived from whey, casein, soy, pea, rice, and other sources. They can help individuals meet their protein needs, especially post-workout.

Proteins play several critical roles in muscle building:

- **Muscle Repair and Growth**: Proteins are essential for repairing and building muscle tissue after exercise. Resistance training causes micro-tears in muscle fibers, and protein provides the amino acids necessary for repair and growth.

- **Muscle Protein Synthesis (MPS)**: Consuming protein stimulates MPS, the process by which the body builds new muscle proteins. This is crucial for muscle recovery and growth, especially after workouts.

- **Satiety and Weight Management**: Protein is more satiating than carbohydrates or fats, which can help control appetite and support weight management. Maintaining a healthy body composition is important for optimal muscle growth.

- **Hormone Production**: Proteins are involved in the production of hormones that regulate various bodily functions, including those related to muscle growth and metabolism.

- **Immune Function**: Proteins play a role in the immune system by forming antibodies that help protect the body against infections and diseases.

General recommendations are:

- **For Muscle Building**: 1.6 to 2.2 grams of protein per kilogram of body weight per day (or about 0.7 to 1 gram per pound).

- **For General Health**: 0.8 grams of protein per kilogram of body weight per day (or about 0.36 grams per pound).

Macronutrient Breakdown Priorities

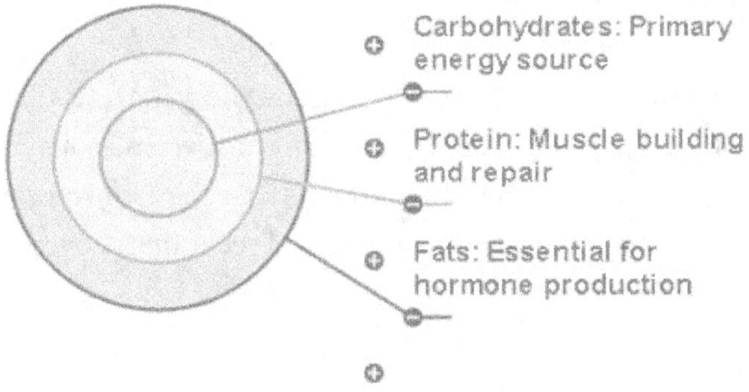

Now let's get to tracking your calories. First, before you start measuring your food on a scale you need to decide how you're going to measure it, whether measuring the food before it's cooked or after it's cooked.

Some people say that measuring it before it's cooked allows you to eat more food. I don't know how true that is. I've always done it after it was cooked and it has worked for me greatly. Whichever one you choose, make sure you keep using that method as that will give you more concrete data and feedback.

If you don't have a scale, make sure you buy one. Or you can buy a meal already done for you by a meal prep company if you have the money for it. It's a great time saver if you're a busy person and dont have time to prepare meals.

There are several apps that you can use to track your calories and macros. The most famous one that I have used for years is MyFitness Pal. But there are other free alternatives in the app store as well. MyFitness Pal lets you track your calories for free but if you want to track your macros as well you'll have to make an investment.

To know your calories and macros, you can go to this website Yillex.com, you put in your age, height, sex, weight, activity level and your goal and it will spit out the calories and macros you need to eat according to your goals. And it's free.

Disclaimer: chances the calories and macros you get are 100% right and that is okay. Tracking calories is not an exact science, maybe the calories you get are too much or too little. If that's the case you can add or decrease 10-20% of your total calories and see if that moves you in the right direction you want to go.

Principle 3: Track your workouts

You need to establish a baseline from what you work on. If you just go into the gym and do whatever comes to mind there's a good chance at some point you will feel stuck. If you're just going to the gym to just workout and feel good then that strategy might work for you.

But if you want to keep moving forward and see what you're capable of then you need to track the exercises that you're doing, the weights, the reps and your tempo.

Remember when we talked about progressive overload? This is a good way to know that you are effectively building muscle and getting stronger as well. Plus, it's fun to lift heavy-ass weights!

Don't worry about being perfect, chances are you are going to suck at first but as long as you have the desire and the work ethic you will make progress.

Principle 4: Take Measurements

Another good way to know if you're making progress, especially if you want a good aesthetic physique is progress pictures. Sometimes it seems like even though we are doing the best we can we are not moving forward so taking pictures is a visual comparison from where you have been and where you are right now.

You probably won't see changes from day-to-day pictures but 8-12 weeksfrom now the changes will be noticeable.

The scale is another way you can measure progress if your goal is weight loss or weight gain.

With that being said, many people fall into the trap of getting their self-worth from the number on the scale. Remember, the number on the scale is just a unit of measure. It doesn't reflect who you are.

Another way you can take measure is to get a measuring tape and measure the circumference of the body part.

Principle 5: Get a Training Partner

You can make a lot of progress quicker if you can get a training partner. That way you can have some friendly competition and motivate each other to keep pushing.

There will come a time that you will need to train past failure and having a training partner is a massive advantage. Now, I'm not saying that you wont make progress if you don't have one, you most definitely can. In my first year of training, I trained all by myself and put on 20 pounds of muscle.

Another great idea would be to hire a personal trainer that works in that gym. Just make sure they know what they are doing.

5

The Role of Supplements

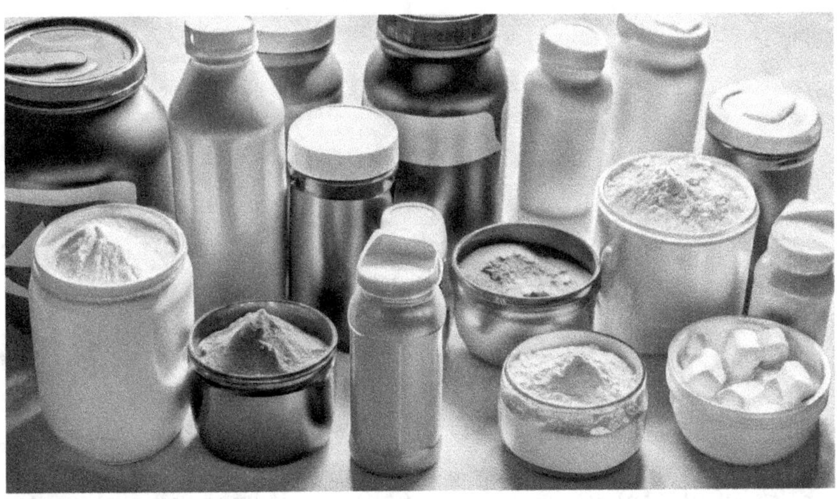

While proper nutrition is the cornerstone of building muscle, supplements can complement your dietary efforts and fill gaps in your intake. Here's a breakdown of essential supplements for beginners and their benefits:

- **Protein Powders:** Protein is key for muscle repair and growth. For those who struggle to meet their protein requirements through food, protein powders like whey or plant-based options (pea, hemp, or soy) can be convenient. They are great post-workout to promote muscle recovery.

- **Creatine Monohydrate**: A well-researched supplement known to improve strength, increase muscle mass, and enhance overall performance during high-intensity workouts. It's safe for most people and should be taken daily, mixed with water or juice.

- **Branched-Chain Amino Acids (BCAAs)**: These are essential amino acids (leucine, isoleucine, and valine) that play a role in muscle recovery, reduce muscle soreness, and support endurance during workouts. They are especially helpful when training fasted or on a calorie deficit.

- **Fish Oil (Omega-3)**: Omega-3 fatty acids improve joint health, reduce inflammation, and aid in overall recovery. This is especially useful since bodybuilding can sometimes cause joint stiffness or pain.

- **Multivitamins**: Although not directly related to muscle building, multivitamins ensure that you meet daily micronutrient needs, which can support energy levels, immune function, and metabolism.

- **Caffeine**: A popular pre-workout ingredient, caffeine enhances focus, reduces fatigue, and boosts performance during workouts. Beginners should assess their tolerance and avoid over-consuming.

Choosing the Right Supplements

It's important to note that supplements are not a substitute for a balanced diet. You should:

- **Research Thoroughly**: Ensure the supplements are from reputable brands and backed by scientific studies.

- **Avoid Over-Reliance**: Use supplements to complement a solid nutrition plan, not as a shortcut.

- **Consult Professionals**: Consult with a dietitian or trainer if unsure about the right supplements for your needs.

Remember, each individual responds differently to supplements, so tracking your progress and tweaking your intake is key.

32

6

Application Suggestions

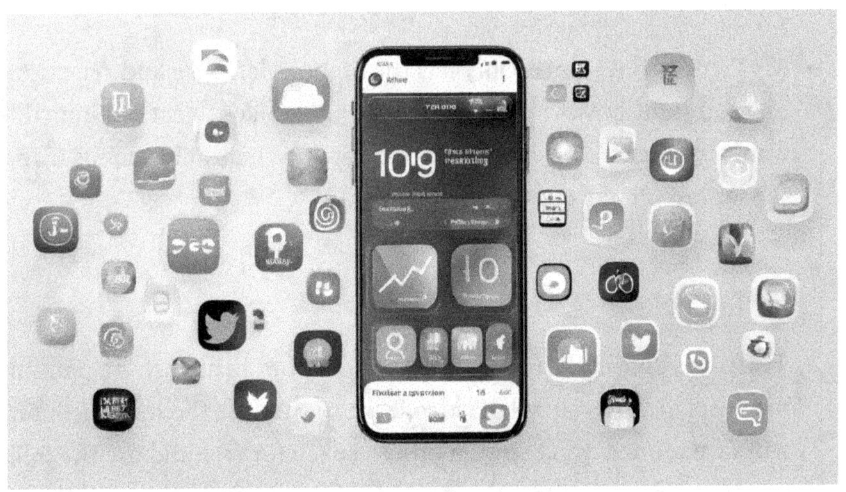

There are some great apps out there that I have used that helped me save time from making my own workouts and my nutrition. I'm not sponsored by them, this is just free game and some hacks that will save you some money.

- **Coachify**: good app for tracking your workouts and nutrition in one place. The biggest con for me is that the exercise selection is not great and it's pretty basic.

- **RP Hypertrophy**: it's a bit expensive, but it's great because depending on the feedback you give it, it will alter your workout program so that you can keep making progress without falling into the usual pitfalls that most people do.

- **MyFitness Pal**: it probably has the biggest database and selection on food right now. If you're somebody that likes to eat out but still wants to stay on track this is a good app for you. It has menus from the largest chains out there.

- **Trainerize**: this is a hack that i thought about using. It's a pain in the butt because you will have to learn how to use the website but it will save money, you can sign up as a coach for free and use the free slot to train yourself, and if you add the nutrition add-on (i think it's $5-$10) you can track your calories and macros. Now you can track your nutrition and workouts for about 5-10 dollars a month.

I'm sure there are other ones out there that are great. Do your research and use the one that works best for you.

7

Understanding Anatomy

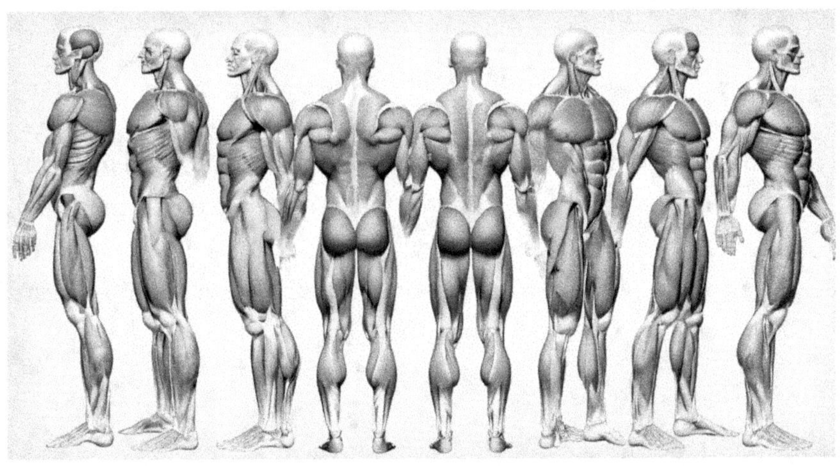

An understanding of muscle anatomy is critical for targeting specific muscle groups during workouts and preventing injuries. Here is an overview of several major muscle groups, including their origins, insertions, and primary functions in movement, along with examples of workouts that effectively target each group:.

- **Quadriceps**: The quadriceps are a group of four muscles located at the front of the thigh. They originate from the pelvis and femur and insert into the tibial tuberosity via the patella. These muscles are responsible for knee extension, a movement primarily engaged during exercises like squats, lunges, and leg presses.

- **Hamstrings**: Found at the back of the thigh, the hamstrings originate at the ischial tuberosity of the pelvis and insert at the tibia and fibula. The hamstrings are critical for knee flexion and hip extension, making them vital for movement like deadlifts, hip thrusts, and sprinting.

- **Gluteals**: Comprising the gluteus maximus, medius, and minimus, these muscles originate from the pelvis and insert onto the femur. They are responsible for hip extension, abduction, and external rotation, activated during movements such as squats, hip thrusts, and step-ups.

- **Pectoralis (Chest Muscles)**: The pectoralis major and minor make up the chest muscles. They originate from the clavicle, sternum, and ribs and insert onto the humerus. They are responsible for shoulder adduction and internal rotation, exercised through chest presses and push-ups.

- **Lats (Latissimus Dorsi)**: These large back muscles originate from the lower spine and pelvis and insert into the humerus. They are critical for shoulder extension, adduction, and internal rotation, as seen during pull-ups and lat pulldowns.

- **Traps (Trapezius)**: Originating from the skull and spinal vertebrae and inserting onto the scapula and clavicle, the trapezius muscle stabilizes and moves the shoulder blades. It plays a key role in exercises like shrugs and overhead presses.

- **Biceps**: Located at the front of the upper arm, the biceps originate from the scapula and insert onto the radius. They are responsible for elbow flexion and forearm supination, engaged during bicep curls and chin-ups.

- **Triceps**: Found at the back of the upper arm, the triceps originate from the scapula and humerus and insert onto the ulna. They are responsible for elbow extension and are worked during tricep dips and overhead extensions.

- **Deltoids (Shoulders)**: These muscles originate from the clavicle and scapula and insert onto the humerus. The deltoids allow for shoulder abduction, flexion, and extension, targeted during lateral raises and presses.

- **Abs (Abdominals)**: The rectus abdominis, obliques, and transverse abdominis originate from the ribs and pelvis, inserting along the midline of the abdomen. They stabilize the core and support spinal movements, exercised through planks, crunches, and leg raises.

- **Calves**: Comprising the gastrocnemius and soleus, these muscle groups originate from the femur and tibia, inserting onto the heel bone via the Achilles tendon. They are crucial for plantarflexion of the ankle and are activated during calf raises and running.

Understanding these muscle groups provides a foundation for optimizing your workout routine and achieving balanced muscle development.

8

Common Injuries and Muscle Recovery Techniques

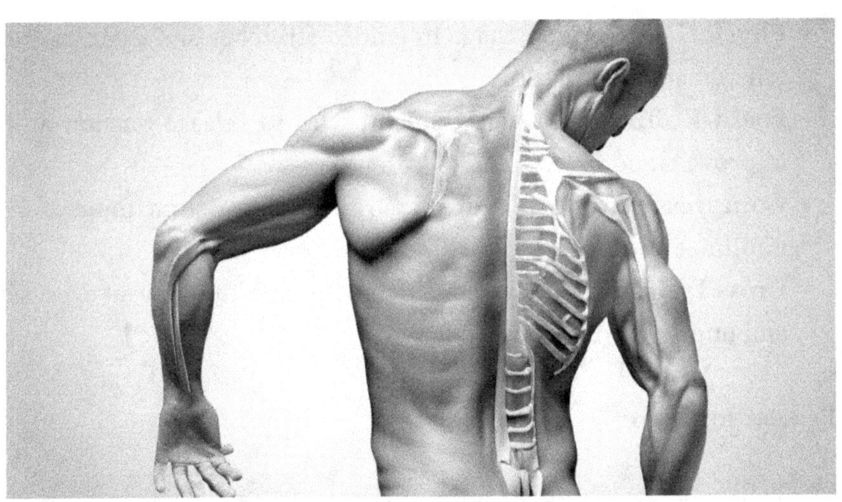

Bodybuilding or strength training, while rewarding, can sometimes lead to injuries if not approached with proper caution. Here are common injuries along with techniques to recover and prevent them:

Common Injuries:

- **Sprains and Strains:** Often caused by improper form or excessive weights.
- **Tendinitis:** Overuse of a particular joint leading to inflammation (e.g., elbow or shoulder).
- **Lower Back Pain:** Frequently due to poor posture during heavy lifts such as deadlifts.
- **Rotator Cuff Injuries:** Straining the shoulder muscles from inadequate warm-ups or poor technique.

Recovery Techniques:

- **Rest and Ice:** Allow the affected area to heal and reduce inflammation.
- **Physical Therapy:** Engage in guided stretches and exercises to rehabilitate injured areas.
- **Foam Rolling:** Massage tight muscles to release tension and improve blood flow.
- **Compression and Elevation:** Especially for joint injuries to minimize swelling.
- **Cross Training:** Incorporate different exercises to prevent overuse and improve overall strength.

Prevention Tips:

- Always warm up thoroughly before exercising and cool down afterward.
- Use proper technique and avoid lifting weights beyond your capacity.
- Incorporate rest days and focus on active recovery.
- Strengthen supporting muscles to stabilize joints and prevent excess stress.

Taking a proactive and planned approach minimizes injury risk and ensures consistent progress in your bodybuilding journey.

9

Essential Gym Equipment

When starting your gym journey, having the right equipment can make your workouts safer and more effective. Here's a guide to essential gym gear:

1. **Weightlifting Belt**:

- Purpose: Provides support for your lower back during heavy lifts such as squats and deadlifts.
- Tip: Use it for sets where you are lifting close to your one-rep max.

1. **Wrist Straps**:

- Purpose: Helps enhance your grip for pulling exercises like deadlifts and pull-ups.
- Tip: Use sparingly to still work on your natural grip strength.

1. **Lifting Shoes**:

- Purpose: Ensures stability and proper posture during weightlifting exercises.

- Tip: Look for shoes with a flat sole or slight heel. You can get squatting shoes that have an elevated heel.

10

Commonly Asked Questions

1. How long does it take to see results in?

- **Answer:** Results vary per individual, but noticeable changes often occur after 8-12 weeks of consistent training and proper nutrition. Beginners may see faster progress due to the body adapting to new stimuli.

2. Do I need to take supplements to build muscle?

- **Answer:** Supplements are not mandatory. Prioritize a well-balanced diet. Supplements like whey protein or creatine can be helpful if dietary needs aren't met.

3. How many days per week should I train?

- **Answer:** Beginners should aim for 3-4 days per week of full-body workouts. More advanced lifters can progress to 4-6 days with split routines.

4. Is cardio necessary for muscle building?

- **Answer:** While not crucial, cardio improves cardiovascular health and complements weight training. Include 1-2 sessions weekly for overall fitness.

5. What should I do if I hit a plateau?

- **Answer:** Evaluate your training, nutrition, and recovery. Strategies include increasing intensity, changing your routine, or boosting calorie intake.

11

12 Week Workout Programs

Full Body Program

Suggested schedule:

- Monday: Full Body
- Tuesday: Rest
- Wednesday: Full Body
- Thursday: Rest
- Friday: Full Body
- Saturday: Rest
- Sunday: Rest

	Exercise			Muscles worked	Rest
Day 1	Barbell Squat	4 sets	6–8 reps	Quads, glutes, hamstrings, core	3-5 minutes
	Barbell Bench Press	4 sets	6–8 reps	Chest, shoulders, triceps	3-5 minutes
	Bent-Over Barbell Row	4 sets	6–8 reps	Back, biceps, rear delts	3-5 minutes
	Dumbbell Lateral Raises	3 sets	12–15 reps	Shoulders (lateral delts)	2-3 minutes
	Barbell Romanian Deadlift (RDL)	3 sets	8–10 reps	Hamstrings, glutes, lower back	2–3 minutes
	Hanging Leg Raises	3 sets	12–15 reps	Core, hip flexors	2-3 minutes
Day 2	Deadlift	4 sets	5–6 reps	Hamstrings, glutes, lower back, traps	3-5 minutes
	Pull-Ups (Weighted if possible)	4 sets	6–8 reps	Lats, biceps, rear delts	3-5 minutes
	Dumbbell Incline Bench Press	4 sets	8–10 reps	Upper chest, shoulders, triceps	3-5 minutes
	Bulgarian Split Squats	3 sets	10–12 reps per leg	Quads, glutes, hamstrings	3-5 minutes
	Dumbbell Hammer Curls	3 sets	10–12 reps	Biceps, brachialis	2-3 minutes
	Plank (Weighted if possible)	3 sets	30–60 seconds	Core, shoulders	2–3 minutes

Day	Exercise	Sets	Reps	Muscles	Rest
Day 3	Overhead Press (Barbell/Dumbbell)	4 sets	6–8 reps	Shoulders, triceps, upper chest	3-5 minutes
	Front Squat	4 sets	8–10 reps	Quads, core, glutes	3-5 minutes
	Dumbbell Chest Fly	3 sets	12–15 reps	Chest (pecs)	3-5 minutes
	Barbell Pendlay Row	4 sets	6–8 reps	Back, biceps, rear delts	3-5 minutes
	Tricep Dips (Weighted if possible)	3 sets	10–12 reps	Triceps, chest, shoulders	2–3 minutes
	Cable Face Pulls	3 sets	12–15 reps	Rear delts, traps, upper back	2–3 minutes
	Russian Twists (Weighted)	3 sets	20 (10 reps per side)	Obliques, core	2–3 minutes

Upper/Lower Program

Suggested schedule:

- Monday: Upper
- Tuesday: Lower
- Wednesday: Rest
- Thursday: Upper
- Friday: Rest
- Saturday: Lower
- Sunday: Rest

12 WEEK WORKOUT PROGRAMS

Day	Exercise	Sets	Reps	Rest Period
Day 1: Upper Body (Push Focus)				
	Barbell Bench Press	4	6-8	3-5 minutes
	Dumbbell Incline Press	3	8-12	2-3 minutes
	Seated Overhead Dumbbell Press	3	8-12	2-3 minutes
	Cable Chest Fly	3	12-15	2-3 minutes
	Dumbbell Lateral Raises	3	12-15	2-3 minutes
	Overhead Dumbbell Tricep Extension	3	10-12	2-3 minutes
	Rope Tricep Pushdowns	3	12-15	2-3 minutes

Day 2: Lower Body (Quad Focus)

Front Squat	4	6-8	3-5 minutes
Bulgarian Split Squats	3	8-12	2-3 minutes
Hack Squat (Machine or Barbell)	3	8-12	3-5 minutes
Step-Ups (Weighted)	3	10-12	2-3 minutes
Leg Extensions	3	12-15	2-3 minutes
Standing Calf Raises	4	15-20	2-3 minutes

Day 3: Upper Body (Pull Focus)

Weighted Pull-Ups or Lat Pulldown	4	6-8	2-3 minutes
Barbell Pendlay Rows	4	6-8	3-5 minutes
Dumbbell Chest-Supported Rows	3	8-12	2-3 minutes
Cable Rear Delt Fly	3	12-15	2-3 minutes
Barbell or Dumbbell Bicep Curls	3	8-12	2-3 minutes
Incline Dumbbell Hammer Curls	3	12-15	2-3 minutes

Day 4: Lower Body
(Hamstring/Glute Focus)

Romanian Deadlifts (RDLs)	4	6-8	3-5 minutes
Barbell Hip Thrusts	4	8-12	3-5 minutes
Dumbbell Step-Through Lunges	3	8-12	2-3 minutes
Glute Kickbacks (Cable or Machine)	3	12-15	2-3 minutes
Lying Hamstring Curls	3	12-15	2-3 minutes
Seated Calf Raises	4	15-20	2-3 minutes

The Infamous Bro Split Program

Suggested schedule:

- Monday: Chest
- Tuesday: Back
- Wednesday: Shoulder
- Thursday: Rest
- Friday: Arms
- Saturday: Legs
- Sunday: Rest

12 WEEK WORKOUT PROGRAMS

Day	Exercise	Sets	Reps	Rest Period
Day 1: Chest				
	Barbell Bench Press	4	6-8	3-5 minutes
	Incline Dumbbell Press	3	8-12	3-5 minutes
	Decline Bench Press (Barbell or Dumbbell)	3	8-12	2-3 minutes
	Cable Chest Fly (High to Low)	3	12-15	2-3 minutes
	Dumbbell Pullover	3	10-12	2-3 minutes
	Push-Ups (Weighted or Bodyweight)	3	12-15	2-3 minutes

Day 2: Back

Deadlifts	4	5-6	3-5 minutes
Pull-Ups (Weighted if able)	4	6-8	3-5 minutes
Barbell Bent-Over Rows	3	8-12	3-5 minutes
Seated Cable Rows	3	10-12	2-3 minutes
Lat Pulldown (Wide Grip)	3	10-12	2-3 minutes
Face Pulls	3	12-15	2-3 minutes

Day 3:
Shoulders

Overhead Barbell Press	4	6-8	3-5 minutes
Arnold Press	3	8-12	3-5 minutes
Dumbbell Lateral Raises	3	12-15	2-3 minutes
Cable Front Raises	3	12-15	2-3 minutes
Rear Delt Fly (Dumbbell or Machine)	3	12-15	2-3 minutes
Dumbbell Shrugs	3	12-15	2-3 minutes

Day 4: Arms

Barbell Bicep Curls	4	8-12	2-3 minutes
Incline Dumbbell Curls	3	10-12	2-3 minutes
Hammer Curls	3	12-15	2-3 minutes
Close-Grip Bench Press	4	8-12	2-3 minutes
Overhead Dumbbell Tricep Extension	3	10-12	2-3 minutes
Rope Tricep Pushdowns	3	12-15	2-3 minutes

Day 5: Legs

Exercise	Sets	Reps	Rest
Barbell Back Squat	4	6-8	3-5 minutes
Romanian Deadlifts (RDLs)	4	8-12	3-5 minutes
Bulgarian Split Squats	3	8-12	2-3 minutes
Leg Press	3	10-12	3-5 minutes
Walking Lunges	3	12-15	2-3 minutes
Standing Calf Raises	4	15-20	2-3 minutes
Seated Calf Raises	4	15-20	2-3 minutes

12

Last Words

I hope you enjoy this and it's helpful to you. Even though this book is about bodybuilding and nutrition, this is more of a journey of self-love and being true to yourself. Yes, bodybuilding is a sport but anybody that goes to the gym to get better are also bodybuilders even if they never compete or see themselves in that light. And honestly, it doesn't matter.

To anybody that picked up this book and made it this far…

Thank you. This is the first book I've ever written and I really appreciate you taking the time to read it.

J.D.

References

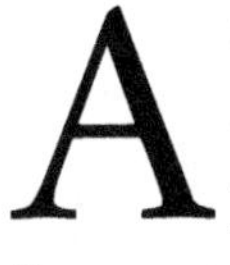

A rapid review of mental and physical health effects of working at home: how do we optimise health? https://bmcpublichealth.biomedcentral.com/articles/10.1186/s12889-020-09875-z

Can Stress Cause Death? https://psychcentral.com/stress/is-stress-the-number-one-killer#how-stress-affects-the-body

Muscle Growth And Sleep Benefits https://working4health.org/nutrition/muscle-growth-and-sleep/

How Sleep Impacts Muscle Growth? https://sleep.me/post/sleep-and-muscle-growth

How the Body Uses Sleep to Bulk Up https://askthescientists.com/sleep-muscle/

The Importance Of Sleep https://www.bodybuilding.com/content/

the-importance-of-sleep.html

Sleep for muscle recovery: Why it matters and tips to sleep better
https://www.betterup.com/blog/sleep-for-muscle-recovery